Natural Treatments for Joint Pain: Making use of Nature's Power to Reduce Pain and Increase Mobility

Copyright © 2023 Tom Pawson

TABLE OF CONTENTS

INTRODUCTION

Welcome to Natural Remedies for Joint Pain, a comprehensive guide on understanding and treating joint pain with the use of nature's healing abilities. This book aims to provide you with a wealth of information, practical tips, and all-natural remedies that can lessen joint pain, promote greater range of motion, and enhance your overall quality of life. This book provides a thorough understanding of joint health, regardless of whether you're seeking supplements or substitutes for your existing medical care.

Pain in one or more joints might affect different body sections. A number of factors, including age, weight, past injuries, overuse, and other medical issues, can contribute to joint pain.

CHAPTER ONE
Understanding Joint Pain

Joint pain: what is it?

Commonly, people have joint stiffness in their hands, feet, hips, knees, or spine. Pain might be intermittent or persistent. The joint may occasionally feel painful, achy, or stiff. A searing, throbbing, or "grating" feeling is reported by some patients. Furthermore, the joint could feel tight in the morning but will become more flexible and comfortable with exercise. Excessive physical exertion, though, may exacerbate the pain.

Pain in the joints might impair their capacity to function and make it harder for them to perform daily duties. Extreme joint discomfort can make living less enjoyable. In addition to addressing pain, treatment should address the activities and functions that are impaired.

Who is more vulnerable to joint pain?

- People with past history of joint health issues. people who overdo or utilize a muscle repetitively.
  Individuals that suffers from chronic illnesses, like arthritis.
  those who experience stress, anxiety, or depression.

People who are obese.

People who experience ill health.

In addition, age has a role in painful and stiff joints. Middle-aged or older persons may experience joint difficulties as a result of years of use and wear and tear.

Let's now discuss the causes of joint pain. The following are the most frequent reasons for persistent joint pain:

A common kind of arthritis called osteoarthritis develops over time when the cartilage, which acts as a cushion between the bones, ages. The joints start to hurt and stiffen. Osteoarthritis typically strikes in middle age and progresses slowly.

Rheumatoid arthritis is a long-term condition that results in joint swelling and discomfort. The joints frequently distort; this mainly affects the fingers and wrists.

Gout is an excruciating disease in which the body's crystals gather in the joint, producing excruciating pain and swelling. Usually, the big toe is affected by this.

overuse-induced bursitis. Usually, the elbow, shoulder, knee, or hip are affected.

A fever, rash, or viral illnesses might cause pain while moving joints.

injuries like sprains or fractured bones

An inflammation of the tendons, which are the flexible bands that join muscle and bone, is known as tendinitis. It commonly results from overuse and is felt in the shoulder, elbow, or heel.

investigating the effects of inflammation on pain and joint health.

Inflamed joints can become painful and swollen. Arthritis and injuries are two possible causes of inflammation in the joints. The underlying cause may affect the course of treatment. The condition may impact a single joint or it may be more systemic, affecting several joints in the body. The body's natural immune response to an injury, infection, or irritation is inflammation. Inflammation can be caused by infections, wounds, and allergies. Injuries and inflammatory arthritis are the most frequent causes of inflammation in the joints. Injuries-related pain and inflammation typically go away, but inflammatory arthritis is a chronic illness that could worsen over time. Chemicals that produce swelling and other symptoms in a joint are released by the immune system or injured tissue, resulting in joint inflammation. One joint may be the only one affected, as in the case of an injury. However, a number of other joint inflammatory episodes can occur throughout the body as a result of specific medical disorders.

The blood arteries surrounding an inflammatory joint widen, enabling more blood to enter the area. White blood cells, an essential component of the immune response, quickly arrive at the site of inflammation and begin combating any infection or irritant.

Inflammation results from this reaction in this region. Inflammation may exacerbate the pain of an underlying injury or infection, and the joint may feel hot or uncomfortable.

Inflammation aids the body's short-term defense against harmful intruders. On the other hand, persistent inflammation may harm the joint.

Identifying risk factors and understanding the importance of early intervention.

There are several factors that can raise someone's risk of developing joint discomfort. While certain conditions cannot be prevented, there are ways to lessen your risk, such as by eating a different diet, giving up smoking, taking good care of your teeth and gums, and taking probiotics. Let's look at the potential causes of joint pain.

Genetic Elements A person may be more susceptible to joint discomfort if a close relative suffers from it on a regular basis. Nonetheless, a variety of hereditary and environmental variables probably play a role. Everybody who experiences joint pain does not have the same genetic mutation causing it.

Hormonal Component Women are two to three times more likely than males to suffer joint illness, according to the Centers for illness Control and Prevention (CDC). Research on the potential involvement of hormones is underway.

The development of female sexual traits is attributed to the steroid hormone known as **estrogen factor**, which is connected to the female reproductive organs. The development of the condition may be aided by high concentrations of estrogen, a female sex hormone that is also found in males. Furthermore, studies have shown that women who have never given birth may be more susceptible to joint disease.

Testosterone Factor Low testosterone levels have been linked to joint problems, according to some research. Researchers released the findings of a 2018 study that included 61 individuals without joint illness and 59 individuals with the ailment who were matched for age and sex. Testosterone levels that were above normal were more common in those with joint illness. Here's an additional factor. Menopause Influence A different research investigation found that certain females with joint illness saw a reduction in physical abilities during and after menopause.

Although **Age factor** joint disease can strike anyone at any age, aging raises the risk. It usually appears in people who are in their 60s.

Factor of Smoking Researchers have discovered connections between smoking and a higher risk dependable source of joint disease development, even in those with chronic, low-level smoking exposure. Smokers may also be more susceptible to severe joint problems.

 Stress Factor: According to study, stress could be a factor in joint illness.

 Research on the **Obesity Factor** has established that obesity raises the risk of joint disease development.

Additional variables include gut flora, nutrition, and a person's history of infection.

the significance of prompt intervention.

The proverb "an ounce of prevention is worth a pound of cure" is perhaps truer in the field of pain management than it is in other areas of medicine. Never dismiss pain, regardless of the source—it could be from an injury, arthritis, a long-term illness, or localized issues like knee and back discomfort. Seeking prompt medical assistance is essential to keeping acute discomfort from turning into a chronic condition that could change one's life. We'll explore the reasons it's imperative to treat pain concerns as soon as possible in this book, as well as the possible repercussions of putting them off.

The Consequences of Ignoring Pain

Consider a situation in which a pain that seems mild is dismissed as the product of a demanding day. You may think it's not worth bothering a doctor about, or you may think it will go away on its own. But even the mildest kind of discomfort might cause other problems in your body.

Physical Restitution:

Your body is a complex network of interdependent parts. Your body may begin to compensate for a painful area by moving other components to lessen the load. For instance, you may inadvertently put greater strain on your right leg if you're favoring your left knee because of discomfort. This may result in an entirely different set of issues.

Emotional Effect:

 Your mental health can suffer if you are in constant discomfort. It may result in poorer quality of life, anxiety, sadness, and sleep difficulties.

Development of Chronic Pain: Ignored pain frequently turns into a chronic problem. A modest discomfort can develop into a chronic illness that is more difficult to manage.

Early Diagnosis Is Essential

Timely diagnosis is the first step towards early intervention. When you speak with a pain management specialist You offer yourself the best opportunity of figuring out the origin of the discomfort at the outset. An early diagnosis enables your doctor to analyze your health more accurately and create a treatment plan that successfully tackles the problem.

For instance, there are a number of reasons why you might be suffering knee pain, including arthritis, overuse, and injuries. Early diagnosis and treatment planning can assist identify the precise reason and let you to start on a personalized course of care that may involve physical therapy, medication, or lifestyle modifications.

Holding Back Progress

The potential to stop pain from getting worse is one of the strongest arguments for early intervention. If left untreated, many acute pain problems might develop into chronic illnesses. Treatments for chronic pain may need to be more aggressive and can be considerably more difficult to manage. For example, conservative measures such as physical therapy and pain medication can typically be utilized to manage back pain resulting from a herniated disc if it is treated quickly. But if neglected, it can result in nerve damage and chronic pain that can need surgery.

Enhanced Life Quality

Prompt action not only keeps pain from getting worse but also makes a big difference in your quality of life. You're making an investment in your wellbeing when you decide to get help for your pain. Without discomfort stopping you, you can carry on with your everyday routines, keep up your mobility, and engage in the activities you enjoy.

CHAPTER TWO: Nourishment for Joint Health

Discovering the key nutrients that support joint health

Even if joint pain is not an issue for you, it is still vital to maintain a balanced diet. However, you might want to include these items in your diet to help with inflammation and joint health if you do suffer from joint pain brought on by osteoarthritis or inflammatory arthritis.

Food treatments may be the solution if you wish to improve overall joint health and reduce inflammation in your joints. Here are some of the best nutrients that reduce inflammation for healthy joints, along with a list of foods that should be avoided that cause inflammation.

Nuts and seeds: Rich in heart-healthy Omega-3 fatty acids, these foods can help lower inflammation in your joints and connective tissue. Almonds, pine nuts, flax seeds, walnuts and chia seeds are good examples under nuts and seeds.

Additionally, **cold water fish** is a great source of omega-3 fatty acids. These nutrients have anti-inflammatory properties and can also reduce the risk of diabetes, heart disease, and other illnesses. You can supplement your diet with fish oil on a daily basis or include fish like halibut, tuna, salmon, or trout.

Fruit: Rich in antioxidants, fruits help relieves joint pain by lowering inflammatory levels in the body. One fruit with potent flavonoids that suppress your body's inflammatory response is blueberries. Bromelain, another potent ingredient found in pineapple, has been demonstrated to reduce joint discomfort associated with osteoarthritis and rheumatoid arthritis. Also in tomatoes an antioxidant Lycopene, helps with issues concerning physical health.

Broccoli, cauliflower, and Brussels sprouts are examples of **cruciferous vegetables**. It has been discovered that these meals inhibit the enzymes that cause joint edema. Additionally, lentils are a fantastic source of vitamins and minerals.

Beans and Pinto: A kind of flavonoid called anthocyanins, which helps lower inflammation in the body, is present in beans, chickpeas, black beans, soybeans, and lentils. Additionally, beans and lentils are an excellent source of fiber, protein, and other minerals.

Olive Oil: Certain oils, such sunflower, vegetable, and peanut oils, might make inflammation worse. On the other hand, olive oil works very well in place of cooking or salad dressings. It is rich in those inflammation-fighting Omega-3 fatty acids and a healthy fat.

Whole Grains: Although the body's inflammatory response can be triggered by the proteins in refined grains, whole grains have the potential to mitigate this effect. Whole rye, barley, whole wheat, and oats are among the grains that are suggested for reducing inflammation and pain in the joints.

Garlic and Aromatic Root Vegetables: The anti-inflammatory qualities of garlic, onions, ginger, and turmeric are well-known. They can be used to treat arthritic symptoms such as joint discomfort. Garlic and root vegetables can be added to meals to improve joint health and add flavor.

Dark Chocolate: Due to the antioxidants in cocoa that fight inflammation, it is delicious and excellent for joint paint. The secret is to indulge in moderation and select chocolate that has a high cocoa content.

The items on the above list are typically included in any diet that promotes health. To maintain a diet that supports bone and joint health, you don't need to look for any unusual items. Even if joint discomfort isn't a constant problem for you, incorporating these foods into your diet is still worthwhile because they offer a host of additional health advantages. Curious in how to maintain the health of your joints? Including items that both prevent and cure joint pain in your diet may be a crucial first step. Making healthy eating a habit is crucial because the things you put in your body have an impact on your overall health. Selecting foods that fortify connective tissue, increase bone density, and reduce inflammation can protect joints, fend off injuries, and provide all-natural relief from joint discomfort.

Avoiding Inflammatory Foods

It's important to know what to avoid in addition to what foods to include in your diet for healthier joints. Certain meals might exacerbate joint pain and internal inflammation. Foods that cause inflammation that you should avoid or limit include:

- prepared meals
  Fried dishes
  Saturated fats or oils rich in Omega-6 fatty acids
  Refined carbohydrates and sugar

investigating the advantages of including foods high in anti-inflammatory properties in your diet.

Your body's response to foreign things, such as chemicals, pollen, and germs (such as bacteria, viruses, and fungus), is inflammation. Although inflammation happens to defend your body, if it persists for an extended period of time, it may begin to negatively affect your health.

Numerous illnesses, including arthritis, cancer, diabetes, and heart disease, are associated with chronic (long-term) inflammation. Your joints may become painful and swollen as a result of persistent inflammation. The tissues that comprise your joints, such as the bones, cartilage, ligaments, tendons, and membranes lining them, can sustain damage over time due to inflammation.

An anti-inflammatory diet: what is it?

An anti-inflammatory diet can help reduce the symptoms of arthritis and/or persistent joint pain. For those who suffer from arthritis or joint pain, there isn't a formal anti-inflammatory diet to follow, but you can manage your inflammation by including some anti-inflammatory items in your meals. On anti-inflammatory diets, fresh fruits and vegetables, whole grains, lean protein, and foods high in omega-3 fatty acids are preferred over processed, fried, and charred meats as well as those high in trans fats. Reduced salt intake is another key component of anti-inflammatory diets; instead, utilize spices and herbs to enhance flavor in your meals and snacks.

How do foods that are anti-inflammatory lessen inflammation?

Some meals, like fried foods, exacerbate inflammation by causing your body to produce more free radicals. Your body's levels of free radicals can also be increased by lifestyle choices like smoking and consuming alcohol, as well as environmental influences like air pollution and pesticides.

Oxidative stress, which destroys your body's cells and is connected to a number of illnesses, including rheumatoid arthritis, is brought on by an excess of free radicals.

Although your body naturally creates antioxidants to combat free radicals, adhering to an anti-inflammatory diet, which includes natural antioxidants, can be beneficial. A diet that reduces inflammation is not a rigid regimen with unbending guidelines. Rather, it is a way of eating that emphasizes the numerous advantages of maintaining a nutritious, well-balanced diet. You may lower the amount of inflammation in your body by eating less inflammatory foods—like fried, processed, high-salt, and high-sugar foods—and more anti-inflammatory foods—like brightly colored fruits and vegetables, dark, leafy greens, fatty salmon, and legumes. Long-term joint health can be achieved by combining this with regular exercise and a balanced lifestyle. Creating a balanced diet that improves general health and lessens joint discomfort is also crucial.

CHAPTER THREE: The Power of Herbal Remedies

Understanding the efficacy and safety of herbal remedies for joint pain, such as turmeric, ginger, Boswellia and devil's claw.

In every culture, people have used herbs for health and healing purposes throughout history, much to how we now drink tea with mint to help with digestion or gargle with garlic to prevent colds. Herbs were the approved forms of medicine when Hippocrates lived. Several herbs are antiviral, antifungal, and antibacterial, and they also contain essential nutrients. Natural plants are still the source of many pharmaceutical medications we use today, and we can still benefit from these natural sources of healthcare.

Let's now examine several herbs that are naturally effective in treating joint pain:

Boswellia: In Asia and Africa, this has been used for generations to relieve pain and inflammation. These days, alternative health professionals commend it for having anti-inflammatory qualities. This herbal extract from the Boswellia serrate tree, also referred to as Indian Frankincense, is believed to function by preventing leukotrienes, which are chemicals that can assault healthy joints in inflammatory illnesses like rheumatoid arthritis. This herbal medicine, which comes in tablets or topical creams, might help cure rheumatoid arthritis and osteoarthritis. It may interfere with or lessen the effects of other medications, so see your doctor first, especially if you are using other painkillers for inflammation.

Turmeric: One of nature's most powerful medicines, curcumin, is what you get when you consume Indian food. Curry recipes call for turmeric, a yellow-orange powder. Turmeric's primary component, curcumin, has been utilized as a food and medicinal for thousands of years in China and India. Turmeric has emerged as one of nature's most potent medicines, according to current studies. The Indianapolis-based Methodist Research Institute notes a "significant anti-inflammatory action." Psoriasis and rheumatoid arthritis are two inflammatory diseases that are relieved by curcumin. Curcumin is a cheap cooking spice that may be added to practically any cooked cuisine, including meats and vegetables, as well as salad dressing. It is essential to take a supplement to receive the greatest results for joint discomfort.

Ginger: In addition to warming and soothing your body, fresh ginger stimulates blood flow to remove toxins and aid in healing. Because the same molecules that give ginger its potent flavor also have anti-inflammatory qualities, ginger is a common ingredient in many cabinets of complementary medicines. As a treatment for osteoporosis, rheumatism, and arthritis, ginger is well-respected. In one study, 18 participants with osteoarthritis and 28 participants with rheumatoid arthritis received three to seven grams of ginger each day from Indian experts. Over 75% of research participants said they had experienced some degree of pain and edema reduction. Discover new ways to savor the fiery flavor of ginger. Fresh ginger can be grated and added to stir fries, tea steeped in ginger, salad dressings, smoothies, and baked goods. Additionally, you can compress arthritic joints with cold ginger tea.

Devil's claw: This has compounds that may reduce edema. It is frequently used to treat illnesses that entail both pain and inflammation as a result. The dried roots of the devil's claw were brought to Europe in the early 1900s and were used to treat pain, inflammation, and heartburn in addition to reviving appetite. Devil's claw is now frequently used in Germany and France to treat low back pain, headaches, and arthritis. It also helps combat inflammation.

Useful advice for introducing herbs into your daily regimen

Natural herb growth dates back thousands of years. They have been used as perfumes, to improve flavor, to treat infections, to cure illness, and to help the body perform its daily tasks. Here are some ideas to start adding herbs into your daily routine if you're looking for new methods to reap all of their advantages.

Cooking (perhaps the simplest): For generations, people have used herbs in their food. You can add it to baked dishes, sautés, soups, salads, and crockpot meals, whether it's fresh or dry. Learn about your herbs by incorporating them into every meal; it may be like a science experiment. Once you know what you're cooking, start combining smell and sight by inhaling the various herbal scents before adding them to your mixture. A small amount goes a long way, and although you cannot take what you have added back, you can always add more. Try new things and don't be scared to "ruin" a dish. It is likely to be well liked even if it is overpowering when combined with a herb like ginger.

As an aside, cook your herbs on low until very last. Herbs can release their taste and health benefits without soaking or cooking for an extended length of time.

Aspirations

Using your own herbs, you may quickly prepare **tinctures** at home. Below is a basic recipe that you can use. Herbs can be incorporated into your body at a concentrated level with tinctures. For someone who doesn't cook for himself often but yet wants to benefit from the wonderful properties of various herbs, this can be a fantastic option. Let's imagine you have a history of inflammation and you've heard great things about turmeric, licorice root, and dandelion. Although you're unsure of how, you can see that these plants may be incorporated to food. A simple and effective way to incorporate them into your system is to make a tincture. All you'll need is a small amount of time, some dried or fresh herbs, an 8 to 16 oz mason jar, a dark dropper bottle, cheesecloth or mesh strainer, vodka, or brandy.

This is a simple recipe: Make use of chopped herbs. Only add 1/2 to 3/4 of the jar to the herb. Fill the jar all the way to the top with alcohol. Cover all of the plants!

Soak for six weeks in a dark, warm storage space. For ease of use, strain and transfer into a dropper bottle.

It is imperative to conduct thorough study on dosages before to use. This is how you are removing all of the plant's nutrients, thus understanding is essential. Additionally, the characteristics of the plant material you're using will determine the proper alcohol strength for your tincture. Not always is stronger better.

Tea

This is an excellent method to truly get to know your herbs and is quite simple to begin with. The most popular method of consuming herbs is through tea, and we have some of the greatest blends for a variety of purposes. To view our list of blends, visit our Tea page. In addition to those amazing teas, we can make a bag of mixed herbs exclusively for you.

Mocktails

A creative and entertaining method to encourage you and your family to drink more water is by making mocktails. They essentially consist of one ice tea and some fruit! Anywhere in your kitchen, you can set up a simple hydration station where you can pause and enjoy herbal-infused drinks throughout the season.

A few fantastic pairings: Basil, peppermint, fresh orange rosemary, fresh lemon serum, and elderflower and fresh lime lemon balm and fresh peach

This is a go-to method for using the incredible advantages of plant therapy. You can extract the plant compounds (the therapeutic characteristics) by steeping your herbs or flowers in specific oils, then apply the resulting form to your skin. Millions of pores on our skin, the biggest organ in the body, allow everything to be absorbed. You can immediately absorb the advantages of a handmade, plant-rich infused serum or lotion into your bloodstream.

As you can see, incorporating herbs into your life may be done in a lot of easy ways. The greatest method to use herbs is just to do it. It may seem overwhelming at first, but start with some staples like making a tincture out of lemon balm and using it in tea. Next, try adding it to your next soup.

Dr Tom Pawson

CHAPTER FOUR: Managing Joint Pain through Essential Oils

Joint pain and inflammation might interfere with day-to-day activities. It is possible to feel better, though. OTC and prescription drugs may be helpful, as well as essential oils derived from plants. The use of essential oils dates back thousands of years. Aromatherapy is the use of them for medical or therapeutic purposes. What you should know is as follows.

How Do Essential Oils Work?

They are a plant's fragrant sections, which are typically the peel, bark, or leaves. When the plant is crushed, you may smell them. Unique steaming techniques also enhance the scent. The smell of essential oils is potent. However, it isn't what makes you feel better. Chemicals in the plant have an impact on your body and mind. When you apply the oil to your skin or breathe it in, they enter your bloodstream.

Essential Oil Types

They are numerous. However, there is scientific proof that suggests certain oils may be able to reduce knee and joint discomfort. They consist of:

Bergamot

Black cumin (Nigella sativa)

cinnamon

Eucalyptus

frankincense and myrrh

Geranium

Ginger

Lavender

Lemongrass

Orange

Rosemary

Peppermint

Aromatherapy is a useful application of essential oils for medical purposes. It might also lessen your perception of pain and tension. To truly understand the benefits of essential oils, more research is required. These are the results of a few modest studies:

black cumin. For three weeks, elderly people used black cumin oil three times a day to their aching knees. Compared to the group that took acetaminophen alone, they felt better.

Eucalyptus: Individuals who inhaled eucalyptus oil experienced reduced pain and blood pressure following total knee replacement.

Myrrh and frankincense: In combination, these oils reduced inflammation in the joints of arthritic rats. Researchers are examining the potential benefits of therapy for ailments including rheumatoid arthritis.

Ginger: Following a ginger oil massage, a group of individuals with persistent knee issues reported less pain and stiffness one month later. Not so did the group that received merely a massage. Additionally, their total physical function was better.

Lavender: Osteoarthritis in the knees and musculoskeletal pain were relieved by a lavender oil massage.

Lemongrass: For thirty days, a small group of rheumatoid arthritis patients who used lemongrass oil reported a slight reduction in discomfort. Citral, a plant molecule, is thought by experts to have anti-inflammatory properties.

Using Essential Oils: A Guide

Avoid applying essential oils straight to your body. It could cause skin irritation or stinging. Here are a few pointers:

Apply massage. Add ten to fifteen drops of essential oil to one ounce, or two tablespoons, of carrier oil. These are oils such as jojoba, avocado, coconut, almond, or olive. That will facilitate absorption and protect your skin. Anywhere you experience joint pain, massage into your skin. Additionally, you can massage some into your neck, wrists, feet, and behind your ears.

Breathing. You can slowly wave an open bottle of essential oil in front of you, apply a few drops on a cloth, or inhale the scent. A waterless or water-based diffuser is another option. That is a device that emits a mist of essential oils into the atmosphere. Observe the dosage recommendations.

Always start with a tiny area of your skin to test. Watch for signs of an allergic reaction. Possible symptoms include:

wheeze or coughing

A rash,

a headache,

And what not to do

The prevailing consensus is that aromatherapy is safe. However, you can't be certain of what you are getting because it is unregulated. It is not necessary for the label to list every ingredient. Avoid using essential oils while pregnant unless your doctor gives the all-clear. Never use them on infants or young children.

Eat or drink nothing of them. Experts disagree about its safety. Also, exercise caution if you go outside. Certain essential oils, such as bergamot, may increase your skin's photosensitivity.

CHAPTER FIVE: Physical Therapies for Joint Pain

Beyond just helping people lose weight, exercise and regular movement also improves their organ, musculoskeletal, and cardiovascular health. Another simple strategy for keeping joints healthy is regular mobility.

Due to Americans' increasingly sedentary lifestyles, recent studies demonstrate the importance of daily movement. It is well known that people tend to overthink the word "exercise," believing they must fit in an hour of exercise at least five days a week, which can feel unattainable or discouraging. However, even a half-hour strolls each day can reduce significant risk factors for common health concerns, including joint-related difficulties.

Strengthening overall and engaging in movement can help avoid joint issues. Although these issues could potentially arise in the future, your best chance is to maintain a healthy diet and engage in regular exercise along with mobility and flexibility exercises.

Imagine your body as a car that gets stopped and rusts if you don't drive it. Our bodies are the same. The mechanism that allows our joints to "release the grease" is movement. Our joints' synovial fluids function somewhat like automotive lubricant; to keep your joints lubricated, you must move them.

Is it Joint Pain?

Any joint may experience problems. Redness, soreness, and swelling in the joints, along with limping, locking of the joint, stiffness, and overall weakness, are possible symptoms.

It can be challenging to self-diagnose joint discomfort, so anyone who believes they may be experiencing joint pain should consult a rehabilitation professional. These experts can aid in locating the source of the issue, recognizing the kind of joint pain and whether it is related to the joints, and suggesting any kind of exercise or therapy regimens to reduce pain in the afflicted areas.

By using a Blood Flow Restriction machine, we can simulate a high-intensity, low-impact workout for patients without putting any stress on their injured joints. The stronger your muscles are, the more the impact of your daily activities will be absorbed by them, relieving the pressure on the joints. Your joints must bear the brunt of weakened muscles.

High repetition, low impact exercises are the greatest for treating joint pain. Limit weight-bearing activities on the painful area and make sure these exercises reduce rather than increase pain.

They shouldn't be simple, but they also shouldn't leave you in such excruciating pain that the next day you can't work safely. You won't do it or stick with it if it hurts. Exercises for your joints that can change your life should be a part of any pain-reduction program.

Age-related natural bone degradation, wear and tear from prior injuries, cancer, and other movement-related disorders can all result in joint discomfort.

The first things someone should try if they have joint discomfort are therapy and a home workout regimen. It's critical to understand that your sorrow won't go away on its own and to act before you reach a point of hopelessness.

Advice for Beginning an Exercise Program Regular movement is like lotion; the more you move, the more natural lubricants your joints receive to keep them healthy and active. The circulation to the muscles and bones is improved by exercise as well.

It's vital to remember that, if done improperly or excessively, exercise can cause joint pain. Make exercise a priority for your general health rather than merely adding it to your routine to lose weight. Hall offered these three pointers for establishing a regular schedule:

As your body gains strength and starts to accept your workouts more and more, start out cautiously and work your way up.

Adopt a well-rounded approach and include in your regimen activities that target your strength, cardiovascular, mobility, and flexibility.

Your body will manage weight on its own if you follow a healthy diet and get regular exercise. Don't worry about losing weight.

This straightforward stretching and strengthening program can help reduce joint pain:

1. Low-Impact Cardio: Walking, swimming, or cycling are examples of low-impact cardio workouts that can assist boost blood flow to the affected areas and improve joint mobility.

- On most days of the week, try to get in at least 30 minutes of moderate aerobic exercise.

2. Mild Joint Movements: - Take a comfortable seat or lie down.

- Go through the range of motion of the afflicted joints slowly and softly.

. As you become more comfortable, progressively expand the range of motion from small starting points.

- For every joint, repeat these motions five to ten times.

3. Strengthening Your Quadriceps: - Assume a sitting position with your feet flat on the floor and your back straight.

. Straighten one leg and slowly raise it to the highest point you can.

- Lower the leg back down after holding it for a little while.

Repeat 10 to 15 times on each leg.

4. Strengthening Your Hamstrings:

- To maintain balance, stand behind a chair or lean on a sturdy object.

Raise one leg straight up in front of you while maintaining a straight knee.

. Bending at the knee, slowly pull your foot back towards your buttocks.

- Hold for a short while before lowering your leg back down gradually.

Repeat 10 to 15 times on each leg.

5. Wall Push-Ups: - Face the wall and place your palms shoulder height down it.

. Retrace a short step while maintaining a straight posture.

. As you lower your chest toward the wall, bend your elbows.

- Return to the starting position by pushing.

Perform ten to fifteen repetitions.

6. Chair Squats: - Place your feet shoulder-width apart in front of a chair.

. Lower yourself toward the chair gradually, bending at the hips and knees.

. After giving the chair a tap with your buttocks, get back up.

Perform ten to fifteen repetitions.

7. Seated Leg Raises: - Place your feet flat on the floor and sit on a chair with your back straight.

   Raise one leg straight up in front of you while maintaining a straight knee.

   . After a little period of time, release your leg.

   Repeat 10 to 15 times on each leg.

8. Ankle Circles: - Place your feet level on the ground while sitting in a chair.

   - Raising one foot off the floor, slowly turn your ankle in a circle.

   - Perform 10 rounds in a clockwise direction, then 10 in a counterclockwise direction.

   . On the opposite ankle, repeat.

Always begin cautiously, and as your body adjusts, progressively increase the duration and intensity of your workouts. It's critical to pay attention to your body and adjust or cease any exercise that hurts or discomforts you. Seeking expert assistance is advised if your joint discomfort continues or gets worse.

CHAPTER SIX: Heat and Cold Therapies

Enhancing blood flow to the affected area is one of the benefits of heat therapy. For stiffness or muscle discomfort, it works well. The use of cold treatment lessens inflammation. When used for recent injuries and discomfort, it is most beneficial.

For anything from inflammation to strained muscles to arthritis, we utilize heating pads or ice packs. For many ailments and accidents, using heat and cold therapy to treat pain can be quite beneficial and reasonably priced.

The difficult aspect is figuring out when to use heat and when to use cold. A single treatment may even incorporate both at times.

Use ice, as a general rule, for any acute pain or injury, as well as swelling and inflammation. If you have tight or sore muscles, use heat.

How does Heat therapy functions?

Heat therapy improves blood flow and circulation by raising the temperature in a specific location. Even a small temperature increase can help reduce pain and improve muscular elasticity in the affected area. Heat treatment helps repair damaged tissue and relax and calm muscles.

Types

Dry heat and wet heat are the two types of heat therapy. The ideal temperature for both forms of heat therapy should be "warm," not "hot."

Heating pads, dry heating packs, and even saunas are examples of sources of dry heat, often known as "conducted heat therapy." Applying this heat is simple.

Sources of moist heat, also referred to as "convection heat," include hot baths, wet heating packs, and steamed towels. It's possible that moist heat works a little better and takes less time to apply.

It is also possible to use professional heat therapy treatments. For example, tendinitis pain can be reduced with the use of heat from an ultrasound.

You have the option of using whole-body, regional, or local heat therapy. For little pain locations, such as a single tense muscle, local treatment works best. If you just want to treat a local injury, you might use a hot water bottle or little heated gel packs. For more extensive pain or stiffness, regional therapy works best and can be accomplished using heat wraps, a large heating pad, or a steam towel. Hot baths and saunas would be examples of whole body treatments.

When to stop using

Heat therapy shouldn't be used in several situations. It could be preferable to employ cold therapy if the affected area is swollen, bruised, or both. Additionally, applying heat therapy to a region with an open wound is not advised.

Due to the increased risk of burns or consequences from heat application, those with specific pre-existing conditions should not utilize heat therapy. Among these prerequisites are:

Diabetes skin irritation

circulatory disorders

multiple sclerosis, deep vein thrombosis (MS)

Consult your doctor before utilizing heat therapy if you have hypertension or heart problems. See your doctor before utilizing a hot tub or sauna if you are expecting.

Using thermal treatment

Unlike cold therapy, which must be used sparingly, heat therapy is frequently most effective when utilized for an extended period of time.

Heat treatment for only 15 to 20 minutes can typically reduce minor stiffness or stress.

Extended heat therapy sessions, such as a warm bath, can be beneficial for moderate to severe pain. These sessions can range anywhere from 30 minutes to two hours.

How does Cold therapy functions?

Cryotherapy is another name for cold therapy. It functions by limiting blood flow to a specific region, which can greatly lessen pain-causing inflammation and swelling, particularly in the vicinity of a joint or tendon. It has the ability to momentarily lower nerve activity, which also lessens discomfort.

Types

The damaged area can be treated with cold treatment in a variety of methods. Options for treatment include

chilled gel packs or ice packs.

coolant spray

ice massage

ice baths

Other forms of cold therapy that are occasionally employed include cryostretching, which combines cold treatment with physical movement and is beneficial for ligament sprains, and cryostretching, which employs cold to lessen muscular spasms during stretching.

Rooms for whole-body cold therapy

When to stop using

Cold treatment should not be used at home by people with sensory impairments that impair their ability to experience certain sensations because they may not be able to tell if harm is being done. This includes diabetes, which can lead to decreased sensitivity and damage to the nerves.

Cold therapy should not be applied to tense joints or muscles.

If your circulation is compromised, you should avoid using cold therapy.

Using cold treatment

Use an ice pack covered in a towel or an ice bath to treat the affected area at home. It is never advisable to put a frozen item straight to the skin since it may harm the tissues and skin. After an injury, start cold treatment as soon as you can.

Apply cold therapy multiple times a day for brief durations of time. To avoid damaging nerves, tissues, or skin, cold therapy should be applied for ten to fifteen minutes at a time, no longer than twenty minutes at a time. For optimal effects, you can raise the afflicted region.

possible dangers from heat treatment

"Warm" temperatures should be used during heat therapy rather than "hot" ones. You risk burning your skin if you utilize heat that is too hot. There's a danger that using heat therapy when you have an illness could make it more likely for the infection to spread. It is not recommended to apply heat directly to a small region, such as using heating packs, for longer than 20 minutes at a time.

Should you see an increase in swelling, discontinue the medication right away.

Make an appointment to visit your doctor if, after a week, heat therapy hasn't helped reduce any pain or discomfort or if the pain gets worse in a matter of days.

Dangers associated with cold therapy

Applying cold therapy too often or too directly can cause damage to skin, tissue, or nerves if you're not careful.

You should speak with your doctor before beginning cold therapy if you have heart or cardiovascular problems.

For 48 hours, if cold therapy hasn't reduced swelling or injury, get in touch with your physician.

The efficiency of the therapy will be greatly increased by knowing when to employ heat therapy and when to utilize cold therapy. In certain cases, both will be necessary. Patients with arthritis, for instance, may apply heat to stiff joints and cold to swell and hurt suddenly.

Stop using either treatment right away if it worsens the pain or discomfort. You can schedule an appointment to talk with your doctor about other treatment choices if the treatment hasn't made much of a difference after using it consistently for a few days.

Additionally, during treatment, it's critical that you notify your doctor if you experience any bruises or changes to your skin.

By increasing blood flow to your body, heating pads may help relieve back pain, heal injured muscles, lessen inflammation, and ease stiffness in your back.

Back stiffness, joint discomfort, and muscle spasms all restrict movement and make it difficult to perform physical tasks. Even while medication has the potential to reduce inflammation, heat therapy is also beneficial for back pain.

This kind of treatment is not brand-new. Actually, it has roots in the sun-therapy practices of the ancient Greeks and Egyptians. Even the Chinese and Japanese used hot springs as a kind of pain relief.

CHAPTER SEVEN: Lifestyle Modifications

Obesity and excess weight impose additional strain on the knees and joints, which can lead to joint pain. Thus, it's critical to maintain a healthy weight to protect your joints and reduce your chance of developing additional issues like osteoarthritis. The most prevalent kind of arthritis is called osteoarthritis, which is characterized by the degeneration of the cartilage at the tips of your bones. This compromises the health of your joints, resulting in discomfort, edema, and limited joint motion. It is widely acknowledged that obesity is a significant risk factor for osteoarthritis, and that risk factor is modifiable. Your knee joints will be under an additional four kilograms of tension for each kilogram of excess weight you carry. Furthermore, regular activities like ascending stairs strain your knees seven times more than your bodyweight does. This demonstrates the significant effect an additional kilogram of weight may have on the health of your joints.

Losing weight is frequently easier said than done, particularly if you have knee discomfort. It's possible that you hurt when you run, bend, or ride a bicycle. If so, the following lifestyle modifications can support your motivation to maintain your weight loss:

Try some light exercise:

Mild exercise benefits your mental health in addition to aiding with weight loss. In addition to being a significant obstacle to weight loss, stress is thought to be a contributing factor in inflammation, which exacerbates knee discomfort.

Begin by going for a daily walk that lasts at least twenty minutes, and then progressively extend it. Swimming is another low-impact workout to think about. Exercise in the water is an excellent choice if you have joint discomfort because it is less taxing on your muscles and joints than other forms of exercise. If you want to incorporate social interaction into your workout regimen, consider enrolling in aqua aerobics lessons.

Other low-impact activities, like yoga and cycling, are excellent for strengthening your muscles and enhancing joint health in addition to burning calories. Look for local courses and organizations if you have trouble staying motivated to exercise; they offer a great way to connect with others who can encourage and assist you to keep on track. To stay hydrated, make sure you drink more water when you work out.

Keep up a nutritious diet

The secret to long-term weight loss and management is incorporating a nutritious diet into your daily routine rather than resorting to crash diets. You can lose weight by including more veggies into your diet and reducing the amount of your portions. Taking water can also be beneficial. This is due to the fact that occasionally your brain may confuse thirst for hunger, in which case drinking water may quench your thirst and alleviate what your brain misinterpreted as a yearning for food. Keep an eye on what you consume; stay away from foods heavy in fat and added sugar, and give up processed foods like takeout, chips, biscuits, and ready meals. Steer clear of sugary beverages, including fruit juice, as it removes the natural fiber from the fruit, leaving behind a high-sugar beverage. Pick recipes that are naturally high in protein and fiber and that make use of fresh ingredients. In addition to being low in calories, fresh fruit and vegetables are also high in fiber, which helps you feel satiated for longer.

Make a plan for maintaining a healthy weight.

To avoid feeling overwhelmed or deterring yourself from exercising, be careful not to take on too much too quickly in your weight loss journey if you intend to lose weight. In order to include food and exercise into your routine over time, try to cultivate a positive relationship with both of them. Maintaining a regular workout schedule helps boost motivation. Consider establishing a new objective for yourself every week, like getting in five more minutes of exercise. Make sure your objectives are reachable and reasonable. On a Sunday, make a weekly plan for your meals and activity; write it all down. This gives your week structure, increasing the likelihood that you will follow through on your strategy. Don't forget to schedule your snacks in addition to your meals. A nutritious snack in the middle of the morning and afternoon can help you stay focused and full of energy; if you prepare your snacks ahead of time, you're less likely to choose bad selections. Don't forget to schedule some downtime. Because there is a connection between your physical and mental well-being, managing your stress will help you maintain focus.

Ergonomic considerations for joint health at home and work.

Your joint may be strained whether you operate from home or in a poorly planned workspace. You can customize any workspace to meet your needs by using these professional recommendations. Adapt your workstation to your unique requirements and any limits resulting from your arthritis. Many of these adjustments can be made when working from home, and they can help avoid the weariness and joint pain that are associated with prolonged periods of inactive posture. The largest issue isn't always sitting down. Rather, it involves staying still for extended periods of time, frequently in an awkward posture like bending forward. People often assume that standing is the reverse of sitting. That's untrue unless you're moving when you stand up. Moving is the true opposite of both sitting still and standing still. Additionally, we should be moving about a lot to prevent fatigue, muscle strain, and pain related to our jobs. Long stretches of inactivity combined with repetitive movements that overwork the same muscles can cause strains in the neck, shoulders, back, hands, wrists, and even legs. Here's how to modify your routines and environment to reduce stress and increase comfort and productivity.

Adapt Your Posture for Comfort

When it comes to preventing strain and stiffness and treating arthritic pain, consider ergonomics. Everything you use, including the chair and keyboard on your computer, should feel comfortable on your body.

Travel frequently

Every twenty to thirty minutes, get up and take a stroll, and develop the habit of regularly shifting positions. Moving and changing positions are the most effective techniques to address pain, stiffness, and exhaustion.

Orient your computer monitor such that you can avoid looking up.

It hurts the neck to tilt your head to look at a screen that is too high. With the exception of large monitors, the top of the screen should be level with the eyes. The center should be around an arm's length away and 15 degrees below your line of sight.

Maintain a straight upper back and relaxed shoulders while sitting. Make frequent checks throughout the day to ensure that your shoulders are not encroaching on your ears. Keep your arms raised. Verify if the armrests on your chair may be adjusted. You can maintain your wrists straight and your fingers relaxed if you position them such that your upper and lower arms make a 90-degree angle.

Set your feet firmly down on the ground. If it is difficult for your feet to reach the floor, use a footrest. Make sure your primary tools are easily accessible. You should always have your phone, calendar, and any other frequently used items close at hand. This prevents you from reaching for them by bending over or putting your body in strange positions.

Selecting the Proper Chair and Additional Equipment. It could be suitable for you to ask for a workplace accommodation if your workplace does not provide a chair that fits your needs or other necessary equipment.

Choose a chair that supports your lumbar area.
Maintaining a balanced sitting posture that isn't strained requires you to mimic the natural curve of your low back. Place your lower back on the back of the chair and tilt your head back so that your spine follows the chair's lumbar curvature. Select a rolling and swiveling chair. Select a swivel chair with wheels for effortless mobility and a five-point base for stability. Look for a chair that fits well. When sitting back in the chair, there should be a minimum of one inch between the backs of your knees and the seat's edge. Your hips and thighs should be at least an inch broader than the seat of the chair. The back of the chair should be sufficiently broad to support your back without limiting your arm movements. Before you buy, try it. Before choosing one, visit stores and sit in a variety of chairs.

Adjust how your chair fits.

A chair should include levers that are conveniently reachable and adjustable for armrest positions, backrest height and tilt, seat height, and seat tilt. Please take a nap. Shoulder and neck tension can be lessened using headrests.

Put up a holder for documents. There's no need to lean toward the desk because it brings the items to eye level.

Lift up that laptop.

Laptop risers assist in lowering the screen to eye level. For that task, you'll need a second keyboard that can be adjusted to the right height.

Don a headgear.

By doing this, you'll be able to avoid the strain that comes with constantly reaching for your phone or holding it between your ear and shoulder.

Use a mouse and keyboard that are ergonomic.

These are intended to maintain a more neutral posture for the hands and forearms. For instance, vertical mice place and hold your hand in an erect, neutral posture. If you suffer from carpal tunnel syndrome, which is a compression of the carpal nerve in the wrist occasionally brought on by repeated hand and finger movements, these might be helpful. Symptoms of carpal tunnel syndrome include burning, tingling, weak, or numb fingers and wrists.

The role that relaxation and stress reduction strategies play in treating joint pain.

Describe tension. The body's and mind's response to daily stresses and strains is referred to as stress. An excessive amount of stress can worsen pain and increase a person's risk of heart disease and other ailments as well as mental health issues.

Arthritis and stress

Excessive stress can also make it more difficult for those with arthritis to deal with the additional issues brought on by their condition. These issues could include future-focused worries, drug side effects, medical costs, and lifestyle adjustments. You can lessen your discomfort, feel better, and be more capable of handling the additional demands of your illness by developing constructive coping mechanisms for stress. These explanations highlight the significance of stress management in the treatment of arthritis. Acquiring the ability to control stress or deal with it constructively is a skill. Just like any other skill, practice is necessary.

The first explanation of this material is how stressful experiences affect the body and psyche. After that, a stress management program is described.

An inevitable aspect of life is stress. Numerous events in life can cause stress, including moving to a new place, changing careers, getting married or divorced, having a child, or losing a loved one. It can also be frustrating to try to provide for necessities like a roof over your head and food to eat.

Anxiety and long-term illness

The same types of stress that everyone else experiences also affect those who have arthritis. But occasionally, having a chronic illness might cause additional issues. Individuals with arthritis could grow increasingly reliant on their loved ones and medical providers. They might also need to adjust to shifts in their energy levels, interests, jobs, or body image. All of these changes can be distressing and none of them are simple.

In response to stress

Your muscles stiffen up when you're stressed. This can exacerbate your pain due to tense muscles. Depression and stress-related discomfort can spiral out of control. But you can contribute to ending that cycle if you learn how to manage your stress.

Certain bodily responses to stress are predictable. The body swiftly releases substances into the blood during stressful moments. This initiates a sequence of physiological alterations. These include elevated blood pressure, accelerated respiration and pulse rate, and heightened tenseness in the muscles. When stress is managed constructively, the body heals and undoes the harm the stress has produced. Nonetheless, the majority of the time, people don't handle stress well. As a result, tension brought on by stress accumulates and damages the body if left unchecked.

Stress affects the mind in a way that is more unpredictable. These psychological responses differ based on the individual and the circumstance. Feelings of worry, anxiety, aggravation, exasperation, or fury are possible examples. People can perform at their best on stage, in an athletic event, or at an exam when they are under a little bit of stress. People who are under too much stress may become prone to accidents, make many blunders, and lose their ability to function. Stress is like a string on a violin. There won't be any music if the string is too loose (not enough stress). The string will break if it is very taut or stressed. Stress of some kind is required for optimal operation.

Recognize that people react to situations and experiences differently. Some people enjoy having a lot of activities and being busy. Some folks might favor a reduced level of activity and a calmer pace. Something that calms one individual could cause stress in another.

Stress indicators and symptoms

Understanding stress's warning signals and symptoms is the first step toward managing it.

fatigue or exhaustion

tense muscles

Unease

Disturbances

Unease or trembling

Lack of sleep

icy, perspiring hands

appetite loss or rise

clenching jaws and grinding teeth

Common physical problems include fatigue, lightheadedness, headaches, stomachaches, and back or muscular aches.

Some of these symptoms could be brought on by illnesses other than stress, such the flu. Concerning symptoms that persist longer than a week, consult your physician. Should your physician determine that stress is the issue, you can collaborate to comprehend and alleviate it.

Make the most of your tension.

Making stress work for you rather than against you is the secret to effective stress management. Three components make up a comprehensive stress management program:

Find out how to handle stress;

- **Acknowledge the things you cannot alter**

Discover how to combat the negative consequences of stress.

Determine the sources of stress

What worries and concerns you the most? In what circumstances do you feel scared, frightened, or anxious? Determine whether or not you can make changes to the stressful parts of your life after you are aware of them.

Keep a "stress diary" to document stressful situations in your life. Note any physical symptoms that you experience. Try some of the stress-reduction techniques our program suggests and let us know if they were helpful. You'll quickly discover what irritates you the most and the greatest coping mechanisms. Then make an effort to stop those things from happening. For instance, if significant family gatherings typically cause you anxiety, schedule additional sleep in advance to improve your ability to handle the situation.

Express your feelings and ideas.

Discussing your worries with someone is usually beneficial. Maybe someone from your family, friends, coworkers, or the clergy can help you view your issues differently.

Recognize when you are unable to perform a given task.

It's necessary to say "no" to people, and you shouldn't feel bad about it. Refusing additional responsibilities, even for a brief while, could help you feel less stressed.

Be mindful of your time and energy limitations.

If you don't, you can get so exhausted that you can't fulfill your goals as a parent, friend, or lover.

Recognize that you are free to choose whether or not to talk about your arthritis. It might be OK to bring up arthritis if it prevents you from doing certain things. If not, your arthritis is a personal issue.

Learn how to let your anger and other bad feelings out without causing harm to other people. It's acceptable to feel furious! Instead of saying "you are making me angry," try saying "I'm feeling angry." This allows you to express your anger without placing the blame elsewhere. Any verbal "striking" of another individual will simply make them feel attacked. This may make it more difficult to settle the dispute. Gaining the ability to communicate your emotions can help you strengthen your bonds with the people who matter most to you.

Steer clear of depression.

Depression can be brought on by an ailment like arthritis. You might experience melancholy or a "blue" mood, or you might seriously consider giving up and giving in. Depression can worsen your discomfort and make you feel uncomfortable. You can be upset or feel sorry for yourself, wondering "why me?" or "why are other people able to do things I can't do?" The knowledge that these are typical emotions experienced by arthritics may be helpful.

Whether you are sad usually depends on how you handle real or imagined events in your life. You most likely won't take any action to get over your sadness if you think of yourself as its helpless victim. Acknowledge that your emotions are entirely your own fault. You're more inclined to actively work on lifting your mood if you understand that you control your mental state.

Make your life easier.

Examine your actions. Select the most valuable ones and leave out the less valuable ones. Numerous jobs or errands could appear essential. Still, are they? They might only have significance to you. When you're well-rested and in good health, your loved ones cherish you more. Consequently, avoid burning out from attempting to do too much. Do a few things well instead. Furthermore, when you need assistance, ask for it and receive it with gratitude. To make your daily duties easier, you can also use tools and equipment.

Control your time and use less energy.

On days when you're feeling good, it's normal to work harder because you typically experience pain and low energy. Organize each day the night before or first thing in the morning rather than burning out attempting to complete it all. Aim to complete the hardest or most demanding task first thing in the morning. Make time for relaxation breaks and don't forget to take them before you're exhausted. Take it slow and work on big tasks before moving on to lighter ones. Try not to take on too many demanding tasks in one day.

Establish objectives

Setting and achieving goals provides motivation and a sense of accomplishment. Establish attainable short-term goals and take each day as it comes. Don't forget to mention friends and hobbies. Due of the unpredictability of your arthritis, be accommodating when estimating the time required to do a task. Think on your long-term objectives for a while. What changes have occurred in your life since you last considered your objectives? Has arthritis impacted them for you? Right now, what matters most to you? What goals do you have in mind?

Don't use drugs or alcohol.

Recognize that booze and drugs can't make your issues go away. Stress tends to increase a smoker's cigarette consumption. Some people try to escape or solve their issues in life by using drugs, alcohol, or marijuana, among other substances. These drugs will only make your health issues worse. They don't aid in stress management. In actuality, they may eventually make you feel more stressed.

Try to remain well.

Keep in mind that your arthritis is just one aspect of your overall health. People can become so consumed with managing their arthritis that they neglect other aspects of their well-being. For instance, you manage your attitude, exercise routine, and food. You can enhance your energy level, stress level, and mental and physical condition of fitness by reaching your maximum potential.

Make time to have fun and laugh.

Make time for play and engage in enjoyable things that bring you joy. Laughter has a certain something nearly magical about it. No matter how depressed you are, laughing can lift your spirits. You can't be "uptight" and laugh at the same time—laughing releases tension! Laugh with pals or watch a humorous film. You are aware of who you are; follow your pleasure.

Let's talk about rest now.

One of the most crucial things you can do to positively manage stress is to learn how to relax. There's more to relaxation than just lounging back and being silent. Calming the body and mind is an active process that is involved in relaxation. Just like learning to ride a bicycle, relaxing is a skill that requires practice. Knowing how to do something makes it "second nature."

Remember that there is no one correct technique to unwind. What matters is what works for you. Here are some recommendations. Experiment until you identify one or two preferred approaches.

methods for relaxation

First, make an effort to schedule some time in a peaceful location away from people, TVs, radios, and other distractions. Shut the eyes. Tension in the stiff muscles should be released gradually. Sit in a comfortable chair with your feet on the floor and your arms by your sides. Start with your feet and work your way up to your neck. Shut the eyes. Breathe in, telling yourself, "I am," and exhale, saying, "I am relaxed." Keep breathing slowly and silently, telling yourself, for example, that your hands are warm, your feet are warm, your forehead is cool, your breathing is deep and smooth, your heartbeat is steady and calm, and that you are happy and at peace.

For a few minutes, light a candle and concentrate your attention on the flame. After that, close your eyes and focus on the flame image for a minute or two.

Visualize a white cloud moving in your direction. It encircles your suffering and tension. A breeze then appears. It lifts the cloud, carrying your suffering and anxiety with it.

Consider a location where you have experienced happiness or comfort in the past. Try to picture it as precisely as you can, including how it feels, looks, smells, and sounds. Remember all of the good things that happened to you during that time. Give no space to painful or negative ideas.

Picture yourself packing all of your anxieties, pains, and fears into a balloon filled with helium. Now release the balloon and see its disappearance.

Sometimes it helps to just "go on vacation" and let your thoughts wander. These are some recommendations. Make up your own!

Take in a sunset.

Remove your shoes and stroll across the lawn.

On a warm, sunny day, sit in a park and listen to the birds.

Take a seat in front of the fireplace's fire.

Stare at aquarium fish.

Overcoming obstacles to rest

You have to genuinely desire to learn how to relax in order to get over obstacles. The following are a few typical "stumbling blocks" to relaxation:

Guilt for taking a break from your hectic schedule

being ridiculed by other people

being unable to pause and take a moment

Concern for "loss of control."

Keep in mind that unwinding will enable you to better manage the expectations placed upon you. You'll be able to do more and have more fun if you set aside time for leisure later.

It could occasionally feel impossible to take a break and unwind. Because you're too busy to unwind, you can find yourself in a rut or tense. If this occurs, begin as soon as you can, wherever you are. In case you're stuck in traffic, inhale deeply and gradually release the air. Take a little break at the snack bar or restroom lounge if you're at work. Shut your eyes, take deep breaths, and concentrate only on your breathing. Take note of the stiff muscles in your body, such as your shoulders, neck, or forehead, and release them.

More calming advice

Practice for at least fifteen minutes each day. It takes a lot of repetition to make a new habit feel like it's ingrained in you.

Select your preferred techniques. Use your imagination. Recall that there's no one ideal approach to unwind.

When you can, try to fit in quick relaxation breaks throughout the day. Try practicing very basic techniques for even a minute or two, such deep breathing.

CHAPTER EIGHT: Supplements for Joint Health

Find out which vitamins and supplements can help relieve the symptoms of arthritis and what dangers some may provide. Numerous dietary supplements have demonstrated potential in mitigating pain, stiffness, and other symptoms associated with arthritis. Researchers have researched a variety of natural items for joint health, including curcumin, omega-3 fatty acids, SAM-e, and glucosamine and chondroitin. Some of these cures may provide relief from arthritic symptoms, particularly when used in conjunction with conventional treatments. Here is the research supporting the efficacy of some of the most widely used supplements for joint health.

Chondroitin and Glucosamine

When it comes to supplements, glucosamine and chondroitin are two of the most popular ones. They are parts of cartilage, which is the material that cushions joints.

Due in part to different study methodologies and supplement kinds, there has been inconsistent research on these supplements. In individuals with knee osteoarthritis (OA), glucosamine and chondroitin, either alone or in combination with an NSAID and a placebo, were compared in the GAIT trial, a sizable National

Institutes of Health study. While glucosamine helped with pain and function, it wasn't significantly better than a placebo. However, an international trial conducted in 2016 discovered that the combination was just as successful in lowering knee OA pain, stiffness, and swelling.

Research on the best beneficial form of supplements has also varied. According to certain research, glucosamine sulfate works best. For some, glucosamine hydrochloride works better. According to a study that contrasted the two methods head-to-head, they provided similar levels of pain relief.

Fish oil

Fish contains polyunsaturated omega-3 fatty acids, which have strong anti-inflammatory effects. Since inflammation is the primary cause of rheumatoid arthritis, omega-3 fats appear to be more effective in treating it than osteoarthritis. According to a 2017 systematic review of research, taking omega-3 supplements lowered RA-related joint discomfort, stiffness, and swelling. Some people may be able to reduce their need of painkillers and avoid the negative effects by taking these supplements. It could be wiser to turn to the vitamins rather than the ibuprofen in mild cases of arthritis. Omega-3s can also be found in plant-based foods like chia seeds and flax seeds.

SAM-e

The body naturally produces SAM-e, or S-adenosyl-methionine, which possesses anti-inflammatory, cartilage-protecting, and analgesic properties. It relieved joint pain in studies just as well as ibuprofen and celecoxib, but without any of the negative side effects.

Curcumin

The key ingredient in turmeric, the spice with a yellow hue that is a mainstay in Indian curries, is called curcumin. It functions as a potent anti-inflammatory in the body by inhibiting the same enzyme that causes inflammation that celecoxib, a medication that blocks COX-2 inhibitors, does. A daily dose of 1,500 mg of curcumin extract was found to be as beneficial as 1,200 mg of ibuprofen in a research involving 367 individuals with OA of the knee, without any gastrointestinal side effects. Additionally, it seems that this supplement reduces RA discomfort and edema. The body finds curcumin difficult to absorb, which is one of its drawbacks. It is best to consume it alongside a fat source. A significant portion of the supplements will have an oil base.

Additionally, black pepper boosts absorption. Piperine, an extract from black pepper, is added to several supplements. On the other hand, piperine may damage the liver, and it can make drugs more effective by enhancing their absorption, such as carbamazepine (Tegretol) and phenytoin (Dilantin).

Vitamin E

Numerous vitamins, including the antioxidant vitamins A, C, and E as well as vitamins D and K, have been investigated in relation to arthritis. Antioxidant vitamin supplementation has not been shown to alleviate arthritic symptoms to date, however eating a diet high in these elements is generally healthful. Vitamin K plays a role in cartilage development, and both vitamins D and K are crucial for strong bones. If you are lacking in these two nutrients, taking supplements could be beneficial.

Additional Dangers

Supplements are generally safe as long as you take them as prescribed and under your doctor's supervision. However, despite their "natural" designation, supplements may have negative effects or conflict with prescription drugs. High-dose fish oil supplements, for instance, have the potential to thin the blood and interfere with anticoagulant medications like warfarin (Coumadin).

It is possible to consume too much at times, particularly when it comes to vitamins. Certain vitamins, such as B and C, dissolve in water. That implies that your body will eliminate any excess that you take in. However, the accumulation of fat-soluble vitamins, including A, D, E, and K, can be hazardous to your health, so talk to your doctor about appropriate dosages.

Finally, the Food and Drug Administration (FDA) does not subject supplements to the same stringent approval procedures as medications. Every pharmaceutical must undergo an evaluation and approval process by the FDA to ensure its efficacy and safety. It's possible that the ingredients of a supplement are different from what's indicated on the label.

How to Safely Take Supplements

If you decide to try supplements, do so in addition to your arthritis medications—don't use them in place of them. The only treatment that has been shown to decrease joint deterioration is medicine, which they should never replace.

Before taking any new supplement, be sure you're taking the recommended dosage and that it's appropriate for you by consulting your doctor. If a customer anticipates taking a lot of supplements, I do advise them to either invest in a [membership with] an independent testing business like Consumer Labs and check with their physician or find an integrative physician who can assist them. Together with your pharmacist, go over your whole list of supplements and medications to look for any potential interactions.

CHAPTER NINE: Integrating Traditional and Modern Medicine

Joint pain can make daily living difficult and uncomfortable. Arthritis affects millions of people worldwide and is one of the leading causes of disability. Symptoms can range from stiffness in the knees to joint pain that makes it difficult to walk long distances or climb stairs and the need for physical therapy exercises to strengthen the muscles around the knees to adopting lifestyle modifications, including weight loss, to manage symptoms. It is crucial that people with arthritis seek out efficient treatment and high-quality medical care in order to control their condition.

The functions of medical professionals in the management of joint health

Orthopedic surgeons are vital when it comes to managing joint discomfort. They are experts in the identification, management, and surgical procedures required to treat musculoskeletal disorders. In order to provide patients with the finest care and relief from joint pain and arthritis, orthopedic surgeons use a variety of techniques.

Assessment and Diagnosis:

A correct diagnosis is necessary for efficient treatment. Comprehensive evaluations are carried out by orthopedic surgeons, who also undertake physical examinations, MRIs, X-rays, and blood tests in addition to analyzing the patient's medical history. This comprehensive assessment evaluates the degree of joint injury or inflammation and aids in identifying the nature and severity of the ailment.

Non-invasive therapies: When treating arthritis and joint discomfort, orthopedic surgeons frequently turn to non-surgical therapies first. To control pain, reduce inflammation, and limit the progression of disease, these therapies may involve prescribing medicine such as pain relievers, nonsteroidal anti-inflammatory medications (NSAIDs), or disease-modifying antirheumatic drugs (DMARDs). Furthermore, intra-articular.

Herbal medicines, especially when combined with conventional therapies, may help reduce pain and inflammation related to joint health. You should be aware that in addition to using the herbal remedies we covered in earlier chapters, you should also seek modern medical attention if necessary or if the pain is too severe. However, it is highly likely that both can be used in conjunction with one another for maximum benefit.

knowing when to get help and advice from professionals.

Keep an eye out for the following possible indications of joint health:

One or more joints experiencing pain, edema, or stiffness.

reddish-colored or heated joints.

pain or stiffness in the joints.

Having trouble performing daily tasks or moving a joint.

You're concerned about joint symptoms.

joint pain that does not go away after three days.

multiple bouts of joint pain in a single month

Which Kind of Healthcare Professional to Consult

Making an appointment with your primary care physician is a wise first step if you're experiencing joint issues that need to be taken seriously. However, diagnosing arthritis can be challenging at times. You may have to consult a professional. Rheumatologists are experts in conditions pertaining to the bones, muscles, and joints, including arthritis. They are skilled in treating all forms of arthritis, particularly those that need sophisticated care, and in making challenging diagnosis. If you have a specific kind of degenerative arthritis, you might be recommended to see an orthopedist.

Following an Arthritis Diagnosis, you can receive education about your daily arthritis management and medication schedule from a nurse educator or other health care provider who specializes in arthritis. These medical specialists can also point you in the direction of beneficial resources, like those offered by the Arthritis Foundation, which include contacts in the area and information on arthritis and daily living.

CONCLUSION

I commend you for starting this path toward natural joint pain management. Now that you have read Natural Remedies for Joint Pain, you have a toolset of options to assist relieve pain and support joint health in general. Never forget to take care of yourself, pay attention to your body, and seek medical advice when necessary. Accepting the restorative power of nature can help you take control of your joint health and lead a more comfortable and satisfying life. Cheers to many more pain-free and active days!